Biography

Mairead James grew up in Newbridge, Kildare. She attended Liberties College in Bull Alley, Dublin in 2003.
She has two children, Layla and Jai, with her partner, Paul.
The Natural Wellness Book is her first book.

THE NATURAL WELLNESS BOOK

By

Mairead James

Dedication

This book is dedicated to my husband and children, without whom I would not have embarked on the wellness/mindfulness journey.

Also, to James Egan, my mentor, my friend and without whom you would not be reading this book.

INTRODUCTION

Becoming a mother kick-started a passion for wellness, happiness and peace of mind. An urge was sparked to learn how to maintain everyday health and wellness within my family.

I have studied many natural health and wellness methods, and have obtained several different levels of qualifications in natural health and wellness approaches, such as a Pilates trainer diploma, an Alsemia healing certification, as well as gaining a decade of holistic, nutritional natural health knowledge and practice.

It is my desire to make these approaches accessible to everyone, without them having to break the bank on expensive courses, consultants or tutors.

Contents

Section 2: Ailment Index

Section 3: Simple Recipes

THE CONCEPT

Every day we see a mish-mash of articles and news pieces about diabetes, Alzheimer's, cancer, M.S., etc. We also see a sea of natural wellness ambassadors, claiming their way is the way to keep well, promising that if you pay lots of money and follow their regime, that you will essentially have eternal youth, beauty and wellness.

We all want to be well, to be happy, to be comfortable financially, and I am here to tell you that, through years of extensive research, I have found that, for the most part, these approaches being advertised come down to one thing - YOU. Your willingness and desire to be happy and well.

In this busy world, we forget ourselves. We forget that, just as the deer seeks out an arnica plant to eat when injured or a chamomile plant when ill, we too have naturally occurring instincts. If we simply pay attention to ourselves, to our bodies, we can begin to see the reactions our well-being has to the foods we eat, the environments we frequent and the thoughts that we think.

An important thing to remember is that sometimes, even with the best of nutrition, with proper rest and sound mind, the body can still fall ill, so do not count this as a failure. This is completely normal, to get a cold or flu from time to time, it is a natural occurrence which allows the immune system to practice its fighting skills. I am not saying modern medicine should be ignored either. It most certainly should not. The trick is to support the body at all times with nutrition, exercise and mindfulness, so that when illness does occur, the immune system is strong and supported enough to combat the ailment as it is supposed to.

This may sound like a huge undertaking but I can tell you from experience that it is simple in many ways, and as difficult as you make it. This principle can actually be applied to many things.

Mindfulness, as mentioned above, is simply observing yourself. Watching how your body reacts to exercise or lack thereof, how your digestive system functions after different foods, how your emotions react to situations, how your mind reacts to thoughts. Even just reading this concept will have hopefully sparked an automatic observation of yourself already.

If not, just take a moment right now to sit quietly and watch the thoughts flow through your mind. Nothing spectacular may happen, but you realize that your thoughts are just a happening, in the same way as a burp! The thought, the burp, the itch, everything just happens, and there is a choice of how to react.

The same can be said for nutrition; the bodily functions happen naturally, and with awareness and observation, you will notice connections between eating a specific food stuff and how the digestive system behaves, how your bowels move, even how your energy and mood is affected. It really only takes a little moment here and there to stop, be silent and look inward to see what's going on.

Finally, we have exercise. This is definitely an area that is daunting for some people, including myself. I like to have an even-paced lifestyle, relatively calm, so I personally do not want a fitness regime worthy of a gymnast or a body builder. I do not wish to push my body to any extremes, I had enough of that during labor thank you very much. I want a nice, gentle form of exercise that will support the natural functions of my body, strengthen and support my muscles and get the blood flowing, without unnecessarily pushing beyond my limits.

The fitness system I find most fitting for this is Pilates, and that is what led me to study the trainers course. Pilates is a series of gentle stretches, which realign the spine and strengthen muscle function. Don't worry about obtaining a gym membership. It is easy to practice at home.

Pilates also encourages good nutrition and mindfulness alongside these gentle exercises for a complete wellness regime.

My advice then is to incorporate mild exercise into your daily life; partake in gentle stretches from head-to-toe before getting into bed and after waking in the morning. Three minutes is all you need. Take brisk strolls daily or take up swimming. Pick a non-arduous form of exercise that is enjoyable to you personally. That way, it will not feel like a chore to maintain.

Joseph Pilates was a holistic advocate, stating, "With body, mind and spirit functioning perfectly as a coordinated whole, what else could reasonably be expected of her than an active, alert, disciplined person." That's a holistic sentiment right there.

He also said, "First you purposefully acquire complete control of your body and then, through proper repetition of Contrology exercises, you gradually and progressively acquire that natural rhythm and coordination associated with all your subconscious activities."

This guy was born in the late 1800s! What amazingly enlightened forward-thinking he had even in that era.

You may have noticed in this quote he says "Contrology." This was his name for Pilates.

So, why Pilates instead of yoga, or cardio, or other types of exercise? Quite simply, Pilates is an exercise that is accessible to everyone; men and women, young or old, fit or unfit, pregnant, or infirm. It is a full body system, conditioning both body and mind to maximize the precision of muscle control, strength and flexibility in a balanced sequence. It strives for quality of movement rather than quantity, creating body awareness, stamina and coordination.

Some of the Contrology exercises can be performed with the use of mechanisms, which Joseph

Pilates devised originally while in an internment camp, to assure that everyone in his cell block could exercise daily, even the bedridden. He believed that nature has simple laws of life, in terms of coordinated mental and physical health, and by respecting these laws, we can prevent things such as early death through heart disease, cancer, and other ailments caused from unhealthy living.

So that is why I choose Pilates above all other exercise. It is non-strenuous and made specifically to avoid causing further damage. It is easy to execute and promotes spinal health which encourages top quality blood flow.

Pilates himself also believed it is vital to nurture balance from birth.

But many infants are exposed to imbalanced factors from a young age. Here are several examples -

1. Being fed artificial milk instead of nursing milk.
2. Being fed processed foods instead of whole/natural/organic foods.
3. Being overdressed when the child is not cold.
4. Being forced to eat when the child is not hungry.
5. Being sent to bed when the child is not tired.
6. Being made to sit still when the child is overly active.
7. Being made to be active when the child is relaxed.

8. Encouraged to stand and walk too early, unable to sufficiently support his or her own weight.

9. Made to study when the child is clearly disinterested.

10. Being misinformed deliberately to avoid the truth (parents tend to do this with "uncomfortable" subjects.)

11. Led to believe success is measured by acquisition of wealth.

Now, you may or may not agree with all of these sentiments, but honestly everything this man says rings true with me. Children have a natural sense of balance. We adults also have this natural sense of balance, but unfortunately our societal way of life does not always allow for this, or so we believe.

We as adults can try to follow our own natural balance by bringing healthy food with us when we leave home so we can snack when hunger arrives, rather than waiting until meal time. You will find your eating habits are not disrupted, and your weight and mood will balance out.

And by allocating several moments throughout the day (they only need to last 2-5 minutes) where you simply stop, breathe, and stand strong, and observe how you feel, you can alleviate your stress to an unbelievable level.

As parents, we can try to be child-led as much as possible, rather than trying to fit the child into our busy schedule.

If you are a stay-at-home parent, try not to worry about chores or the mess the children create. Enjoy your child while they are young. These moments are fleeting. Nurse on demand, comfort when they are upset, celebrate joy, play, create art and create a mess!

Working parents should try to do the same in the evening. The chores can wait. If you follow your child, you will have moments of head-melting chaos because children are full of energy. But honestly, if your full attention is with the child, your day becomes much easier. They are satisfied and fulfilled.

You would think this leaves no time for you but a content child is a confident child and a confident child is an independent child, so by the time they can walk, they will happily entertain themselves for periods of time with their own imaginative play with siblings, toys, art supplies, etc., thus leaving you a few moments to wash the dishes, shower, study your course, read your book, cook, or just relax.

Pilates has taught me to do what is comfortable in the moment. If my back, neck, or hips hurt, I stretch it out.

If the chores seem like a mountainous task, I do something that seems easier until a moment arrives until the original task seems manageable.

It works. By going with the flow, you become less stressed and everything feels easier to approach.

Within the parameters of holistic, emotion must be tended to. If stress, sadness, anger, worry occurs, this is natural. When an emotion arises for you or your child, question it.

Look at it. Where is it originating? How can it be changed? Asking these questions is better than being overcome by emotion.

If you or your child do become overwhelmed, allow yourselves to have these observations afterwards. All of these things are inspired by my knowledge of Pilates regime and I am eternally grateful to him for creating it. I will not share any exercises in this book as I feel it is vital to learn with a trainer present, to assure correct posturing and prevent damage due to getting it wrong on your own in your sitting room reading directions!

In this book, I am going to share my favorite nutritional tips that I have found over the years. The book is divided into sections.

The first section is a list of my 55 favorite healthy foods and their functions. This will help you learn how to support the body during different ailments at home.

The second section is a simple go-to guide of ailments. When an ailment occurs, you can easily look up the ailment and find a ready-made corresponding list of specific foods to heal your body.

Finally, I will include a recipe section; a small selection of my favorite and simple, recipes to help you get started on the healthy eating road.

Hopefully this handbook will help you on your own path to wellness

Read on and be well!

Mairead
~~~~

SECTION 1:
THE PURPOSE OF HEALTHY FOODS

1. Aloe Vera:

- Antioxidant
- Supports metabolism
- Anti-inflammatory
- Rich in calcium
- Large amount of amino acids and fatty acids
- Natural adaptogen
- Helps with digestion
- Laxative
- Alkalizes the body
- Lowers cholesterol
- Combats skin wounds
- Anti-septic
- Anti-fungal
- Anti-microbial
- Effective against normal burns and sunburn
- Reduces dental plaque
- Reinforces immune system

2. Apple:

- Antioxidant
- Anti-cancer
- Curbs pancreatic cancer by 23%
- Break down gallstones
- Anti-viral
- Phenolic compound in apple skin prevents cholesterol from building in artery walls
- Women are 28% less likely to develop type 2 diabetes if they consume an apple daily
- Stimulates the production of saliva, which reduces tooth decay
- Bowel cleanser
- Avert hemorrhoids
- Keeps diarrhea and constipation at bay
- Protects against Parkinson's

3. Arnica (Tea/Cream):

- Anti-inflammatory
- Rejuvenates scalp
- Cleanses the excess oil and sebum from the head, reducing dandruff
- Stimulates hair follicles
- Prevents split ends
- Slows down premature grey hair
- Carbonic acid and flavonoids are beneficial to your skin
- Reduces the appearance of stretch marks (especially if they are pregnancy-related)
- Heals arthritis
- Effective after tonsillitis surgery
- Promotes healing for bruises, sprains, wounds, broken bones, and even frost bite
- Supports immune system

4. Asparagus:

- Alleviates gout
- Expectorant (breaks down phlegm)
- Glutathione slows down aging and "cellular rust"
- Excellent combatant against cancer of the bladder, breast, colon, lung, prostate, and ovaries
- Folate is essential for cellular division. Effective for pregnant women to prevent birth defects (especially spina bifida) in the fetus
- Vitamin K maintains bone strength
- Diuretic combats PMS related water retention
- Asparagine amino acid fights against rheumatism
- Fights throat infection
- Stimulates kidney functions

5. Avocado:

- Anti-cancer
- Anti-arthritic
- Reduces side effects from chemotherapy
- Inhibits the growth of prostate cancer cells
- Lutein is essential for eye health
- Low in saturated fat
- More potassium than a banana
- Contains absolutely no sodium
- Balances cholesterol
- Perfect alkaline/acid balance
- Fiber feeds good bacteria in the intestine
- Lowers triglyceride levels
- Loaded with monounsaturated fatty acids
- Supports cardiovascular health

6. Banana:

- Blood cleanser
- Removes toxins
- Balances cholesterol
- Mild laxative
- High levels of tryptophan, which is converted into serotonin
- Pectin aids digestion
- Natural antacid that provide relief from acid reflux
- Doesn't exasperate stomach ulcers like most fruits
- Relieve anemia
- Proven by the FDA to lower blood pressure and protect against heart attacks and strokes
- Counteracts calcium loss during urination
- Prevents build-up of lactic acid at night
- Natural antibiotic
- Promotes good sleep

7. Beans:

- Lower blood pressure
- Lowers triglyceride levels which reduces the chances of suffering a heart attack
- Great for people with a sensitivity to gluten
- Balances cholesterol
- Full of iron, copper, phosphorus, magnesium, and zinc
- Contains no cholesterol
- Contains only 2/3% fat
- Packed full of protein
- Metabolized more efficiently than other complex carbs
- Regulates colon and bowel functions
- Antioxidant
- Abundance of fiber
- Anti-cancer
- Keeps blood glucose stable

8.Blueberries:

- Reduces symptoms of diabetes
- Balances glucose
- Maintain brain function and memory
- Anthocyanins lower the risk of a heart attack
- Anti-adhesives prevent bacteria like E. coli from binding to the wall of the bladder
- Reduces muscle damage after strenuous exercise
- Fights against urinary tract infections
- Lipoproteins (bad cholesterol) is oxidized
- Has the highest antioxidant capacity of all commonly consumed fruit and vegetables
- Reduces DNA damage
- Supports bone density
- Lowers blood pressure
- Boosts immune system

9. Broccoli:

- Acids are processed into the anti-cancer compound, sulforaphane
- Supports bowl functions
- Large amount of magnesium and calcium neutralizes blood pressure
- Carotenoid lutein prevents age-related macular degeneration and cataracts
- Eases the discomfort of the common cold
- Prevents the arteries from thickening
- High level of calcium and Vitamin K can prevent osteoporosis
- Glucoraphanin detoxifies and repairs skin
- Supports kidney functions

10. Brown Rice:

- Rich in selenium, which reduces the risk of arthritis and cancer
- Synthesizes fats
- Alleviates diarrhea
- Prevents build-up of arterial plaque
- Regular intake reduces the risk of developing diabetes by 60%
- Excellent baby food
- Perfect adjunct for candida yeast infection treatment
- Releases sugar slowly
- Prevents toxins attaching to the colon wall
- Antioxidant
- Reduce heart disease
- Promotes weight loss
- Naturally-occurring oils normalizes cholesterol levels
- Rice water relieves colic

11. Brussels Sprouts:

- Antioxidant against cellular rust, atherosclerosis, strokes and heart disease
- Glucosinolates fight cancer
- Glucobrassicin reduces inflammation
- Isothiocyanate sulforaphane supports the cardiovascular system
- Prevents hypertension
- Fights lead toxicity
- Combat cataracts
- Maintains low blood sugar
- Protects stomach lining by obstructing the overgrowth of bacteria
- Drastically reduces the risk of gastric cancer
- Compounds block sulphotransferase enzymes from damaging DNA
- Supports immune system
- Anti-bacterial for the gut

12. Cabbage:

- Anti-bacterial
- Anti-cancer
- Indole-3-carbonile is a powerful antioxidant
- Effective against skin eruptions such as eczema, psoriasis, acne, rashes, insect bites, leg ulcers, and wounds.
- Cabbage juice filled with Vitamin D
- Sulfur protects against dried skin
- Strengthens hair
- Stimulates hair growth
- Raw cabbage prevents hair loss
- Vitamin E improves skin complexion
- Filled with Vitamin K and anthocyanins which boost mental function
- Detoxifies stomach, liver and colon when eaten raw
- Supports immune system

13. Cashew Nuts:

- Relieves depression
- Anti-fatigue
- Palmitoleic acids prevent heart problems
- Copper strengthens hair
- Calcium and magnesium strengthens bones
- Keeps blood vessels and muscles relaxed
- Niacin prevents dermatitis
- Zea-xanthin improves the eyes
- Pyridoxine prevents anemia.
- Daily intake of cashew nuts reduces the risk of gallstones by 25%
- Maintains healthy teeth
- Strengthens gums
- Zinc improves gonadal function
- Improves nucleic acid synthesis
- Promotes digestive health

14. Cauliflower:

- Anti-cancer
- Anti-inflammatory
- Antioxidant
- High level of phosphorus and potassium
- Contains 77% of daily value of Vitamin C
- Eating half a cup of cauliflower per day reduces the risk of prostate cancer by 52%
- Fixes damaged cells in the inner lining of the arteries
- Improves cerebrovascular function
- Improves cardiovascular system
- Low in calories
- Reduces the risk of stroke and heart disease
- Promotes digestive health
- Improves blood pressure
- Supports kidney function
- Helps develop the brain of the fetus while it is in the womb

15. Cayenne Pepper:

- Anti-cancer
- Effective against stomach ulcers
- Lowers cholesterol
- Combats sore throat
- Works against diarrhea
- Alleviates spasmodic and irritating coughs
- Anti-bacterial
- Anti-fungal
- Migraine relief
- Allergy relief
- Produces saliva
- Capsaicin is a good joint-pain reliever
- Useful against blood clots
- Boosts metabolic rate
- Excellent remedy for toothache
- Combats gum disease
- Can treat snake bites
- Effective against rheumatism
- Bowel cleanser
- Binds and cleans minor wounds

16. Celery:

- Anti-cancer
- Anti-inflammatory
- Soothes nervous system
- Lipid-lowering properties fight saturated fats
- Prevents degeneration of vision
- Only contains 10 calories
- Stress relief
- Contains good salts
- Vitamin A prevents age-related degeneration of vision
- Reduces bad cholesterol
- Pheromones boost your arousal levels
- Luteolin inhibits the growth of cancer cells
- Regulates alkaline/acid
- Prevents dehydration
- Aids digestive health
- Anti-arthritic
- Lower blood pressure

17. Chamomile Oil:

- Mixing it with Evening Primrose oil handles inflammation
- Eases skin rashes and scarring
- Anti-arthritic
- Anti-cancer
- Anti-dandruff
- Natural antidepressant
- Antioxidant
- Analgesic that offers quick relief against headaches, colds, sinusitis and migraine
- Effective against diarrhea, constipation and gallstones
- Maintains the central nervous system
- Boosts immune system
- German chamomile oil is effective against sciatica
- Neutralizes blood pressure

18. Chamomile Tea:

- Promotes sleep
- Treats cuts and wounds
- Boosts immune system
- Helps with hyperglycemia and diabetes
- Extremely effective against burns
- Anti-bacterial
- Calms muscle spasms
- Soothes stomach ache
- Promotes sleep
- Helps irritable bowel syndrome
- Natural hemorrhoid treatment
- Maintains healthy skin
- Non-caffeinated herb
- Alleviates depression
- Fights against colds
- Alleviates menstrual cramps
- Calms upset stomach

19. Chickpeas:

- Aid weight loss
- Prevents anemia
- Improves diabetes glucose control
- Garbanzos are full of manganese
- Stabilizes blood sugar and low glycemic index (GI)
- Lowers LDL (bad) cholesterol
- Antioxidant
- Saponins fights breast cancer
- Phytochemicals protect women against osteoporosis
- The homocysteine amino acid strengthens blood vessels
- Improves lipid levels
- Improves insulin levels
- Minimizes hot-flushes in post-menopausal women
- Supports connective tissue strength

20. Chocolate (Dark):

- Has more antioxidants than almost any other food
- Balances blood pressure and circulation
- Good for new mothers and babies
- Lowers the risk of suffering from strokes in men
- Balances cholesterol
- Protects arteries near the heart
- Reduce insulin resistance
- Protects lipoproteins against oxidative damage
- Lowers the risk of cardiovascular disease
- Lowers the risk of calcified plaque
- Flavonoids protect against sun-induced damage
- Theobromine improves brain function
- Decreases oxidized bad cholesterol in men
- Promotes cardiovascular health

21.Coconut Oil:

- Lowers cholesterol
- Supports digestion
- Liver cleanser
- Lauric acid boosts metabolism
- Fat burner
- Anti-bacterial
- Antioxidant
- Improves insulin levels
- Helps skin heal faster
- Gets rid of cellulite
- Anti-aging facial moisturizer
- Increase absorption of calcium and magnesium
- Anti-viral
- Fights infection
- Hair conditioner
- Moisturizer
- Dental health
- Regulates thyroid functionality
- Treats candida/thrush
- Supports vaginal health

22. Coriander (Cilantro):

- Lowers cholesterol
- Prevents anemia
- Supports menstrual functions
- Improves diabetes glucose control
- Reduces pimples
- Facilitates hair growth
- Remedy for the cold and the flu
- Anti-diabetic
- Anti-bacterial
- Effective against eczema, itchy skin, rashes and inflammation
- Treats conjunctivitis (pink eye) and other eye problems
- Alleviates nausea
- Supports digestive health

23. Cranberries:

- Anti-bacterial
- Urinary tract cleanser
- Stops breast cancer cells from multiplying
- Supports bladder function
- Fights heart disease
- Citric acid prevents kidney stones
- Fixes bladder problems
- Effective against gingivitis, gum disease, cavities and plaque build-up
- Anti-aging properties
- Promotes weight loss
- Relieves stress, anxiety and depression
- Relieves skin conditions like psoriasis, acne, dermatitis and eczema
- Prevents the clogging of the arterial walls
- Supports intestinal health

24. Echinacea (Tea, Cream etc.):

- Immune system booster
- Urinary tract cleanser
- Promotes healing
- Anti-inflammatory
- Fights bronchitis
- Quells stomach ache
- Echinacea cuts the chances of catching a common cold by 58%
- Reduces the duration of the common cold by 36 hours
- Relieves pain from gonorrhea, measles and bowels
- Effective against rheumatoid arthritis
- Natural laxative
- Effective against brain cancer
- Pain reliever after tonsillitis surgery
- Clears yeast infections
- Calms hay fever

25. Fennel:

- Relieves intestinal cramps
- Keeps neurological diseases at bay
- Absorbs cholesterol
- Oil compounds assist in digestive, carminative and antioxidant reactions in the body
- Enhances the production of red blood cells
- Fat burner
- Stimulates secretion of digestive juices
- Removes more toxic substances during urination than usual
- Releases endorphins
- Prevents macular degeneration of eyes
- Maintain blood pressure
- Abundance of Vitamin A, B, C and E prevent cell damage
- Reverses anemia
- Anti-spasmodic

26. Garlic:

- Anti-bacterial
- Anti-spasmodic
- Anti-viral
- Ant-oxidants that can prevent from Alzheimer's disease and dementia
- Longevity
- Increases estrogen in females
- Minimizes bone loss
- Reduces lead levels in blood by 19%
- Combats osteoarthritis
- Relieves headaches
- Improves athletic performance
- Reduces exercise-related fatigue
- Effective against colds
- Combats hypertension
- Decongestant
- Lowers cholesterol
- Natural antibiotic

27. Ginger:

- Natural antibiotic
- Anti-spasmodic
- Anti-viral
- Chromium, magnesium, and zinc improve blood flow
- Prevents chills
- Combats fever
- Inhibits fatty deposits from the arteries
- Remedies motion sickness
- Improves absorption of water
- Produces cell death in ovarian cancer cells
- Cold and flu prevention
- Fights stomach discomfort
- Prevents colon cancer
- Anti-inflammatory
- Removes mucus and expands lungs, which fights most respiratory problems
- Alleviates excessive sweat
- Alleviates nausea
- Alleviates menstrual cramps

28. Grapefruit:

- Anti-arthritic
- Neutralizes blood pressure
- Very low in calories
- Blocks absorption of carbohydrates
- High in enzymes which cuts down fat
- Low in sodium
- High in water
- Increases metabolism
- Flavanoids keeps the body free from carcinogens
- Blood cleanser
- Pectin works as a bulk laxative
- Protects the colon mucus membrane
- Effective against lung cancer and oral cancer
- Fights throat infection
- Anti-viral
- Lycopene is a powerful agent against tumors
- Anti-bacterial

29. Grapes:

- The resveratrol and proanthocyanidins are effective antioxidants against ultra-violet rays, making grapes effective against sunburn when placed directly on the burnt away for 30 minutes
- Anti-cancer
- Anti-inflammatory
- Anti-histamine
- Combats uneven skin tone
- Helps lighten scars (especially acne scars)
- Colon cleanser
- Keeps skin supple
- Promotes heart health
- Imparts shine to limp, brittle hair
- Helps dissolve kidney stones
- Lowers blood pressure
- Improves diabetes glucose control

30. Honey:

- Natural antibiotic
- Supports immune system
- Flavanoid antioxidants prevent heart disease
- Anti-cancer
- Reduces ulcers
- Fights against bacterial gastroenteritis
- Bees add an enzyme that makes hydrogen peroxide, making honey an anti-bacterial and anti-fungal remedy
- Lowers cholesterol
- Glycogen improves recovery time from athletic activities
- Reduces cough and throat irritation as effectively as dextromethorphan medicine
- Aids wound healing
- Takes approximately 32,000 years to go off (seriously)
- Aids weight loss

31. Kale:

- Prevents anemia
- Anti-cancer
- The quercetin lowers blood pressure
- Anti-viral
- Kaempferol antioxidant is anti-inflammatory
- Contains the recommended daily dose of Vitamin C
- Contains over twice the recommended daily dose of Vitamin A
- Contains nearly seven times the daily dose of Vitamin K
- Prevents a build-up of bile
- Alleviates depression
- Promotes cardiovascular health
- The only fat it contains is omega-3 fatty acid
- Steamed kale lowers cholesterol

32. Lavender

- Lavender oil is effective against anxiety
- Pain relief
- Alleviates insomnia
- Alleviates headaches
- Promotes gastrointestinal health and relieves indigestion
- Having a bath with lavender petals works against muscle ailments
- Relieves apnea
- Effective against dry skin, acne, eczema, psoriasis, eczema, and other skin ailments
- Maintains strong hair
- Reduces risk of heart disease and strokes
- Prevents the growth of harmful bacteria in gut
- Anti-spasmodic
- Anti-convulsant
- Antiseptic

33. Lemon/Lime:

- Anti-arthritic
- Anti-bacterial
- Anti-viral
- Strengthens immune system
- Limonins support optimal health
- Lime juice effective against cholera
- Cleanses blood
- Combats liver damage
- Have an alkalizing effect in the body to help neutralize excess acid waste
- Stops cellular damage and inflammation
- Contains potent anti-carcinogens that prevent the spread of cancer
- Rich in Vitamin A and C, folic acid, flavonoids, antioxidants and potassium
- Dissolve gallstones
- Heals coughs and colds

34. Lentils:

- Folate supports nervous system
- Aids metabolism
- Synthesizes DNA and RNA
- Maintains structure of red blood cells (especially for a fetus while in the womb)
- Regular consumption of legumes reduces the risk of heart disease
- The niacin maintains the functionality of the immune system
- Stabilizes blood sugar
- A cup of lentils provides 87% of the recommended daily dose of iron
- Improves diabetes glucose control
- Prevents anemia
- Provides minerals for most organs
- Supports connective tissue strength

35. Milk:

- Benefits cardiovascular health
- High in protein
- De-stresser
- Effective against P.M.S.
- Reduces the liver's production of cholesterol
- Works against hypertension
- Effective against respiratory problems
- Combats osteoporosis
- Acts as an antacid
- Vitamin A and B help build good eyesight
- Helps against tooth decay
- Decelerates bone degeneration
- High in zinc, calcium and magnesium
- Exfoliant that maintains smooth skin
- Protects against environmental toxins
- Supports immune system

36. Nettle Tea:

- Anti-arthritic
- Anti-histamine
- Support adrenals
- Strengthens fetus in pregnant women
- Promotes milk production in lactating women
- Relieves menopausal symptoms
- Helps with respiratory tract disease
- Supports the kidneys
- Reduces the risk of prostate cancer
- Stops bleeding
- Promotes a release from uric acid from joints
- Stimulates the lymph system to boost immunity
- Helps with diabetes mellitus
- Helps with menstrual cramps and bloating
- Breaks down kidney stones
- Blood cleanser

37. Olive Oil:

- Antioxidant
- Oleocanthal mimics the effects of ibuprofen, which reduces inflammation
- Squalene and lignin enzymes combat cancer
- Particularly effective against breast cancer
- Regular consumption of olive oil lowers the risk of suffering a stroke by up to 41%
- Reduces the risk of Type 2 diabetes
- Promotes cardiovascular health
- Polyunsaturated fats protect against depression
- Combats postmenopausal osteoporosis
- Filled with monounsaturated fats
- Improves arterial function, especially in the elderly
- Lowers the chances of suffering a heart attack
- Lowers blood pressure

38. Onion:

- Anti-spasmodic
- Anti-arthritic
- Rejuvenation properties on body tissues
- Onion juice can work against certain types of moles
- Raw onions stabilize menstrual cycles
- Great cure for common cold, cough, fever, sore throat, allergies, etc.
- Effective against nose bleeds
- Combats insomnia and other sleeping disorders
- Increases the release of digestion juices
- Onion juice is effective against burnt skin, insect bites and bee stings
- Effective against cancer in the head, neck or colon
- Works against atherosclerosis
- Blood cleanser

39. Orange:

- Phytochemicals fight against cancer of the skin, lungs, breasts, stomach and colon
- Prevents kidney disease
- Mandarin oranges are effective against liver cancer due to high level of Vitamin A compound called carotenoids
- Relieve constipation
- Prevents macular degeneration
- Electrolyte minerals maintain the functionality of the heart
- Soluble fiber lowers cholesterol
- Good against arrhythmia
- Abundance of polyphenols fight viral infections
- Vitamin C protects cells by neutralizing free radicals
- Blood cleanser
- Assists the body with iron absorption

40. Parsley:

- Prevents anemia
- Vitamin K aids in bone health
- Vitamin C is a great immune booster
- Beta carotene helps against free-radical damage
- Combats joint pain
- Contains the recommended daily dose of Vitamin A
- Large amount of calcium, iron and folate
- Oxalates prevent gall bladder problems
- Stops kidney disease
- Anti-inflammatory
- Encourages digestion
- Stops muscles from getting stiff
- Fights the effect of aging
- Compounds inhibit tumor growth
- Slows down aging of cells
- Blood cleanser
- Dissolves kidney stones

41. Pomegranate:

- Destroys cancer cells in the breast, colon and prostate
- Pomegranate juice has three times more antioxidants than red wine or green tea
- Punicalagins works as an anti-inflammatory, especially in the digestive tract
- Combats type 2 diabetes
- Effective against obesity
- Works against Alzheimer's disease
- Prevents heart disease
- Supports immune system
- Supports female reproductive health
- Effective against systolic blood pressure problems
- Counters osteoarthritis
- Blocks enzymes that damages joints
- Promotes cardiovascular health

42. Porridge Oats:

- Boost libido
- Balance testosterone
- Balance estrogen
- Effective against hangovers
- Lowers craving for nicotine
- Of all cereals, porridge has the best proportion of protein
- Slowly releases complex carbohydrates, which allows full concentration to be maintained
- Effective against childhood obesity
- Prevents constipation
- Folic acid effective for pregnant women
- High in Vitamin B6, which fights depression
- Supports bone density
- Supports connective tissue strength
- Can be used to ease rash-induced itches

43. Quinoa:

- Anti-viral
- Supports digestion
- Non-GMO
- Gluten-free
- Quercetin effective against depression
- Kaempferol works against inflammation
- Flavanoids attack cancer cells
- Higher in fiber gram for gram than most grains
- Absorbs water
- Reduces blood sugar levels
- Increases fullness
- Lowers cholesterol
- Helps with weight loss
- Contains large amounts of calcium
- Supports bone density
- Supports connective tissue strength

44. Radishes:

- Anti-cancer
- Expectorant and decongestant
- Anti-viral
- Increases fullness
- Vitamin A, C and K effective against skin disorders
- Strengthens cells in skin, hair and nails
- Prevents fat accumulation
- Helps build muscle
- Anti-microbial
- Anti-bacterial
- Healthy for liver
- Lowers the risk of stomach cancer
- Treats jaundice
- Effective against hypertension
- High in sodium
- Plenty of nutrients for pregnant women
- Boosts metabolism
- Aids digestion

45. Raspberries:

- Expectorant and decongestant
- Low in fat
- Prevent damage to DNA
- Prevents macular degeneration
- Low in calories
- Rich in fiber
- High in folic acid, manganese, copper, magnesium, potassium and iron
- High in Vitamin B and K
- High level of phenolic flavonoids which are effective against neuro-degenerative diseases
- Pelargonids prevent cancer
- Catchins combat inflammation
- Ellagic acid de-ages cells
- Xylitol prevents fluctuations in blood sugar
- Supports female reproductive health
- Alleviates menstrual cramps

46. Raspberry Leaf Tea:

- Expectorant and decongestant
- Alleviates menstrual cramps
- Strengthens the uterine wall while relaxing muscles in the uterus
- Improves implantation and lowers the chances of suffering a miscarriage
- Regulates hormones after menopause
- Beneficial for pre-pregnancy; contains huge amounts of compounds that help the body detoxify extra hormones that may impede conception
- Helps with diarrhea
- Supports female reproductive health
- Helps uterus with post-natal recovery
- Labor inducer/cervix softener, (avoid during pregnancy)

47. Rock/Sea salt:

- Stimulates metabolism
- Alleviates bronchitis
- Alleviates psoriasis
- Vitiligo treatment
- Removes acne scars
- Grows hair faster
- Soothes heartburn
- Improves appetite
- Facilitates cellular absorption of minerals
- Stabilizes blood pressure
- Effective against insect bites
- Remedy for rheumatic pain
- Alleviates herpes
- Consumption of rock salt with lemon juice can eliminate stomach worms
- Controls vomiting
- Works against sinus
- Effective against kidney and bladder stones
- Prescribed as a laxative for digestive disorders

48. Sage:

- Fights infection
- Decongestant
- Antioxidant
- High vitamin content
- Lowers sodium
- Works against gastrointestinal discomfort
- Improves cognitive skills in Alzheimer's sufferers
- Lowers blood glucose
- Effective against hyperlipidemia
- Strengthens muscles, especially for women after childbirth
- Significant amount of carbohydrates and protein
- Anti-fungal
- Anti-microbial
- Loaded with fiber
- Effective against diabetes
- Decreases cholesterol
- Anti-inflammatory

49. Seeds:

- Pumpkins seeds boost the immune system
- Prevent anemia
- Sunflower seeds help lose weight
- One of the few vegetarian sources of complete protein
- Contains all 20 amino acids needed to build calorie-burning muscle
- Maintains bone strength
- Regulates high energy levels
- Controls cholesterol
- Sesame seeds have lignan compounds that fight cancer
- Helps with PMS
- Reduces disease-causing inflammation
- Support intestinal health
- High level of insulin
- High in fiber
- Hemp seeds have high level of omega-3 oil
- Maintains good digestion
- Chia seeds are filled with antioxidants

50. Spinach:

- Enormous amount of iron
- Cooked spinach gives thrice the amount of antioxidant as raw spinach
- Immune system booster
- Phytonutrients have anti-cancer properties
- Works against prostate cancer
- Contains lutein and zeaxanthin, which prevent cataracts
- Lowers hypertension
- Helps with insomnia and other sleep disorders
- Promotes gastrointestinal health
- Folate prevents DNA damage
- Prevents mutations in colon cells
- Rich in Vitamin K, which maintains bone health
- Slows down cell division in stomach and skin cancer cells
- Regulates blood pressure
- Supports connective tissue strength

51. Spirulina:

- Antioxidant that prevents damage to DNA
- Inhibits the production of inflammatory signaling molecules
- Phycocyanin has anti-inflammatory properties
- Lowers LDL and triglyceride levels which can prevent heart disease
- Works against type 2 diabetes
- Works against oral cancer
- Decreases the size of lesions and tumors
- Reduces blood pressure
- Counters chronic kidney disease
- Effective against strokes
- Produces nitric oxide, which helps blood vessels relax and dilate
- Supports immune system
- Energy booster

52. Sweet Potato:

- Anti-inflammatory for the intestine
- Blood cleanser
- Vitamin B6 reduces homocysteine which lessens the likelihood of heart disease
- Good source of Vitamin D, which maintains bone strength
- Produces collagen for the skin, which maintains its elasticity
- Effective against SAD (seasonal affective disorder)
- Provides energy for white blood cell production
- Stress reliever
- Metabolizes protein
- Good source of magnesium
- Necessary for maintaining the functionality of nerves and arteries
- Removes heavy metals in stomach

53. Turmeric:

- Anti-inflammatory
- Anti-arthritic
- Induces cell death in the medulloblastoma (a pediatric brain tumor)
- Induces cell death in an aggressive brain tumor called glioblastomas that is resistant against chemotherapy and radiotherapy
- Slows the growth of existing prostate cancer
- Artery cleanser
- Causes melanoma (skin cancer cells) to commit suicide
- Inhibits leukemia cells from developing, especially in children
- Prevents metastasis (cancer spreading to other organs)
- Supports cardiovascular health

54. Water:

- Hydration (Obviously!)
- Prevents fatigue
- Increases motivation
- Curbs headaches
- Effective against anxiety
- Relieve constipation
- Controls calorie-burning functions
- Effective against kidney stones
- Supports and strengthens muscles
- Prevents spasms in muscles and intestines
- Improves skin health
- Strengthens hair
- Maintain bone density
- Maintains concentration
- Helps break down complex carbohydrates
- Improves bowel function
- Supports kidney and bladder health

55. Yoghurt:

- Improve intestinal functionality
- Regenerates good bacteria
- Repairs muscle tissue
- Vital for cell growth
- Vitamin B12 maintains functionality in the brain
- High level of iodine which can combat thyroid problems
- Large amount of Vitamin B12, riboflavin and zinc boosts body's immune system
- Vitamin A prevents macular degeneration
- Essential for healthy metabolism
- Loaded with calcium
- Large amount of potassium balances the sodium in your body
- Regulates blood pressure
- Stores good bacteria
- Great workout recovery food
- Effective against osteoporosis
- Treats candida/thrush

SECTION 2
AILMENT INDEX

1. Abdominal Cramps:
Apples, fennel, garlic, lavender tea, sweet potato, water
For immediate relief, eat a serving of probiotic yoghurt. Garlic and ginger can be grated into the yoghurt to disguise the taste or mixed together into a smoothie. You can also take the garlic or ginger alone. Simply chop them and take them with water as you would a tablet. Lavender tea brewed with fennel can also relieve symptoms. Add apples and sweet potato to your regular intake to prevent abdominal cramps.

2. Aches:
Cayenne pepper, chamomile tea, garlic, ginger, honey turmeric
For bodily aches, brew a tea of turmeric, ginger and cayenne pepper with lots of honey to soften the taste. This tea can be used for colds, flus, chest infections, sinus infections and throat infections. Add lemon to boost the antibiotic properties.

3. Acne:
Coconut oil, water
Having a nutrient rich diet will eventually balance out any issues that cause skins problems such as acne. To ease symptoms when you have a stress-induced flare up, simply use coconut oil as a moisturizer and drink plenty of extra water.

4. Allergies:

Nettle tea, grapes

For minor allergies, such as hay fever or hive rash (urticarial,) adding nettle tea and grapes can ease symptoms. The used teabags can also be placed on the eyes if they are irritated from hay fever.

5. Amenorrhea
(Abnormal absence of menstruation):

Raspberry leaf tea, pomegranate

Drinking raspberry leaf tea supports female reproductive functions, alleviates cramps and may help amenorrhea sufferers. Pomegranate is known to stimulate and support ovarian function, which may also aid this menstrual disorder.

6. Anemia:

Avocado, chickpeas, parsley, spinach, orange

Avocado is rich in iron and can be eaten raw on toast with a sprinkle of salt and pepper, or added to salad and smoothies.

Chickpeas can be added to salads and hot dishes and they are also rich in iron and protein.

To get the full intake of iron from spinach and parsley, I advise that you eat them raw; either used as salad leaves, or mixed into a smoothie. It is important to accompany all of these food items with a glass of freshly squeezed orange juice, or eat an orange following the meal to help aid the iron absorption.

7. Anxiety:

Lavender tea, chamomile tea

Replacing your regular morning tea or coffee with lavender or chamomile tea for even a couple of days should provide quick relief from symptoms of anxiety.

8. Arthritis:

Avocado, broccoli, cayenne pepper, grapefruit, turmeric

Cayenne pepper and turmeric can be brewed into a tea **(See: Aches)** to alleviate arthritic symptoms. Broccoli and avocado can be added to salads.

Grapefruit is best eaten in a fruit salad, as it can make smoothies and juices taste quite bitter.

9. Asthma:

Rock/sea salt, sage, seeds

To relieve bronchial symptoms of asthma, add the rock/sea salt and sage to boiled water and breath in the steam. Wait until the water is no longer boiling. Place your head over the bowl after the water has cooled a little and breathe in the steam. This will quickly open the airways.

Adding seeds to your diet has been known to lessen the occurrence of asthmatic symptoms. You can add seeds to smoothies, salads, porridge, granola or eat them as snacks in their own right.

10. Birth (After Care):

Raspberry leaf tea

This tea should be avoided in pregnancy as it softens the cervix. After giving birth, raspberry leaf tea and raspberries encourage the shrinking of the uterus to its pre-natal size. This will ease the pain dramatically.

11. Bites:

Coconut oil, Oats, nettle tea

Mixing coconut oil and oats into a paste and rubbing onto bites can diminish the irritation. The anti-histamine quality of nettle tea can relieve the itch of an insect bite.

12. Bladder Infection:

Lemon and lime water

If you are suffering from a bladder infection, half-fill a large jar with chopped lemons and limes, and then fill it with water. Pour it from the jar every time you want a drink, refilling the jar as necessary.

13. Bleeding Gums:

Coconut oil

Regular brushing is a given for oral hygiene and health, but using coconut oil as a mouthwash adds extra healing and replenishing properties. Coconut oil soaks up bacteria and toxins, which speeds up the healing process. Swirl the coconut oil around in your mouth and spit it out as you would a mouthwash.

14. Blood Pressure:

Garlic, whole foods

If you suffer from bouts of high blood pressure but do not take blood-thinning medications, then you might consider eating a raw clove of garlic each morning on an empty stomach. You can crush the clove, then chop it finely before swallowing it with water in one gulp. Garlic has blood-thinning properties so one clove a day can lower blood pressure. However, you should consult your doctor if you are already taking blood pressure medications.

15. Bowel Problems:

Probiotic yoghurt, green veg, oats

Probiotic yoghurt is effective against bowel issues due to containing good gut bacteria.

High fiber foods such as green veg and oats support digestion and bowel health. Adding foods such as porridge, granola, cabbage, kale and Brussels sprouts to your diet can promote and support healthy bowel functions.

16 Bronchitis
(See: Asthma)

17. Bruising:

Arnica cream/tea

From minor to major bruising I advise applying arnica cream or gel topically to the affected area.

Arnica tea can also be consumed alongside leafy greens and citrus fruits. All of these foods support and strengthen the body's innate healing functions.

With major bruising, consult your doctor in case of internal bleeding or clotting.

18. Burns (Minor):

Aloe Vera

Immediately after you have been burnt, run the affected area under a cold tap for 10-20 seconds at a time, taking 10-20 second breaks in-between, until the area feels cooler. Then apply aloe Vera to the burned area, place a paraffin gauze, (which keeps the burn moist) and then cover the gauze with a cotton medical dressing. Do not put cotton dressing directly onto the wound.

Change the dressing two or three times daily. Each time the dressing is changed, steep the wound with rock/sea salt water.

If the burn is larger than an inch squared, it is advised to seek medical attention, especially if the injury is to the hand, foot, neck or face.

19. Calcium Deficiency:

Apples, blackberries, broccoli, orange, spinach, quinoa

Creating a salad with broccoli, spinach, and quinoa is fantastic if you are lacking in calcium. Better yet, have the salad accompanied with a freshly blended apple, blackberry and orange smoothie or pressed juice.

20. Cancer:
Whole foods, fruits, veg, berries, cannabis oil

Take as much raw food as possible in the form of smoothies and soups. Smoothies retain all the fibrous parts of the fruits, veg and seeds. You get optimal nutrition with raw food smoothies. Soup allows you to have a large array of nutritious foods in one sitting, which is necessary for those recovering from cancer. It's easy to make and easy to digest.

However, you must remove refined and artificial sugars as these may accelerate cancerous cell growth.

Cannabis oil is also known to break down cancerous cells, as well as quelling the nausea that comes from chemotherapy and radiotherapy.

21. Candida (Thrush):
Probiotic yoghurt, coconut oil

When you catch thrush early, you can effortlessly treat it by applying yoghurt or coconut oil to the affected area, whether its vaginal, penile, oral, or on the nipples. For oral thrush, you need to eat the yoghurt or oil. For other areas, just slather it on generously.

22. Canker Sores (Mouth Ulcers):
Coconut oil

Applying coconut oil directly onto the canker sore gives immediate relief like no over-the-counter pills or prescription gels I have ever used.

23. Cellulite:
Water, Lemon, Honey
Drinking infused lemon water (half a jar of lemon juice, 1 tbsp. of honey and water) helps break down toxins and fats that build up and create cellulite.

24. Chicken Pox:
Oats, coconut oil, blueberries, Echinacea, nettle tea
When chicken pox occurs, it has to run its course. In severe cases, you may be given topical creams or gels for the rash. You can make the coconut oil and oats paste that I previously mentioned **(See: Bites)** and apply to each of the pox to calm the itch and dry the pox spot. You can also add oats to a bath, which will alleviate the itch. Blueberries and Echinacea tea will give the immune system an added boost to fight off the ailment. The anti-histamine properties of nettle tea can also cool the itch.

25. Cholesterol:
Beans, blueberries, garlic
All kinds of beans help to keep cholesterol levels under control. They can make seriously tasty meals when they are teamed up with the equally cholesterol-friendly garlic.

Blueberries balance cholesterol and make delicious smoothies.

26. Circulation:

Garlic, water

As with blood pressure, garlic has blood-thinning and cleansing qualities that will aid circulation, making it easier for clean blood to travel throughout the body.

27. Colds

Garlic, honey, lemon, cayenne pepper, blueberries, Echinacea

Blueberries and Echinacea provide excellent immune boosting qualities.

28. Cold Sores:

Blueberries, coconut oil, Echinacea

Cold sores are generally caused by a deficiency in the immune system, so indulging in blueberries and Echinacea will help work the virus out of your system efficiently.

Coconut oil can be used as a lip balm, (at all times if wanted,) but especially when cold sores are present. The properties of the coconut oil will promote healing, while preventing cracks from developing in the sores.

29. C.O.P.D

Garlic, cannabis oil

When living with chronic obstructive pulmonary disease, incorporating raw crushed garlic to your daily intake will help keep the lungs clear of infection. Cannabis oil is known to alleviate the symptoms of

C.O.P.D. by opening the bronchial walls, allowing proper intake and distribution of oxygen throughout the body. This, in turn, decreases the fatigue that accompanies this disease.

30. Constipation:
Leafy greens, oats, probiotic yoghurt, water
Leafy greens and oats will provide fiber which will help get things moving. Consuming probiotic yoghurt and water can prevent or alleviate constipation.

31. Convalescence:
Dahl, soups, smoothies, water.
When convalescing from any ailment, you can support your immune system by increasing your intake of soups, smoothies, and water.

Lentil dahl is a great detoxing meal as it has high protein content. In dahl form, it is already broken down for easy absorption.

32. Coughs:
Garlic, Echinacea, honey, rock/sea salt, sage
(See: Colds and Asthma)

33. Cramps:
Turmeric, garlic, ginger, raspberry leaf tea
Raspberry leaf tea provides relief for menstrual cramps. A tea brewed from turmeric, garlic, ginger and honey will provide relief from muscular cramps.

34. Croup:

Rock/sea salt, sage, water

Breathing in steam infused with sea salt and sage can open up the airways, alleviating symptoms of a croup.

35. Cuts:

Aloe Vera, turmeric

If the cut is deep but not enough for a stitch, you should pour turmeric powder on the wound. This will kill any bacteria and bond the wound shut. With large wounds, always consult a doctor.

36. Cystitis:

Lemon water, coconut oil

(See: Bladder Infection)

Coconut oil can be rubbed on the urethral opening, around the vaginal area to relieve burning sensations.

37. Depression:

Chamomile tea, cashew nuts

Chamomile tea works wonders for anxiety, depression and even for overactive minds. Cashew nuts have mood boosting properties and are an ideal snack to keep mood levels balanced.

38. Diabetes:

Beans, blueberries, grapes, leafy greens, lentils

Adding high fiber and high protein foods such as kidney beans, chickpeas, leafy greens and lentils to your regular food intake gives your body the components it needs to produce a regulated level of glucose and insulin. Without these foods, it is more difficult for the body to process sugars efficiently.

Blueberries and grapes also provide glucose control. They taste great in porridge, in a fruit bowl or as a smoothie.

39. Diarrhea:

Apples, brown rice, chamomile tea, oats, probiotic yoghurt
When diarrhea occurs, your appetite may not be up to scratch but it's important to eat the foods that will relieve you as soon as possible.

Luckily, the foods that help this condition are mild on the palate and the stomach. Apples are easy to munch on, and the natural acids will help cleanse your stomach and intestines. Brown rice and porridge oats provide fiber, which is needed to prevent or alleviate bowel functions. The naturally occurring good bacteria will also improve the situation, balancing out any bad bacteria that is present. Chamomile tea has anti-spasmodic properties, which is fantastic at quelling the stomach cramps that usually accompany diarrhea.

40. Digestive Health:

Beans, leafy greens, oats, sweet potato, probiotic yoghurt
Beans, leafy greens, oats, sweet potato, and probiotic yoghurt are vital to healthy digestive functions in

general. If you're feeling sluggish, fatigued after meals, or your metabolism seems slow, up your intake of these foods and you will find that it sorts the problem.

41. Dysmenorrhea (Heavy Period):

Raspberry leaf tea, chamomile tea, turmeric tea

As with amenorrhea, these teas relieve menstrual cramping and regulate menstrual flow. However, if you are experiencing bleeding to the extent that you fill a sanitary towel in an hour, it is advised that you seek medical attention.

42. Ear Ache/Ear Infection:

Garlic, olive oil

Pour a couple of tablespoons of olive oil into a small ramekin.

Then crush a clove of garlic to release the antibiotic properties and add it to the olive oil.

Place the ramekin into a bowl of boiled water. This will heat the oil slightly and infuse the garlic and oil.

Dip a cotton ball into the mixture. After you have insured that there are no rogue bits of garlic stuff in it, place the cotton ball in your ear as you would after inserting ear drops.

43. Eyes:
Used teabags

Eyes can get irritated from hay fever, pet or dust allergies, or something getting stuck in it. One remedy for this is a saline eye bath. I find this awkward and therefore ineffective, and tend to opt for used teabags instead. Placing used, cooled teabags of any kind on your closed eyes, (in the same manner as cucumber during a face mask,) will hydrate the area. This will cool the itch and soak out any rogue particles as the bag dries.

44. Fatigue:
Cashew nuts

If you find yourself working long hours, it feels like you cannot fit in enough sleep. If you find yourself in this predicament, stock up on raw, unroasted cashew nuts. Nuts and seeds are excellent sources of protein, and cashew nuts specifically are quickly absorbed into the system, giving more of an energy boost than sugar-filled energy drinks.

45. Fever:
Cold water, garlic

When a temperature turns into a fever, it can be scary. Some people will suffer more symptoms with a temperature than others. Is the person comfortable? Are they delirious? How conscious are they of their surroundings? Is the temperature moving up and down? Drinking plenty of cold water and removing a layer of clothing may reduce the temperature. If the temperature continues to rise, seek medical attention as overheating is dangerous, especially in children.

46. Flu:
(See: Colds, cough)

47. Fungal Nail Infections:
Clove oil, Eucalyptus oil, tumeric
Aromatherapy has several oils that combat fungal nail infections. However, the ones I find most effective are clove and eucalyptus oils respectively. The ultimate treatment has to be tumeric though!

48. Gallstones:
Apples, lemon and limes
When gallstones occur, there can be a lengthy wait for hospital treatment. In the meantime, eat several green apples daily and drink infused lemon and lime water.

You might find that by the time your appointment day arrives, the gallstones may have been partially or fully dissolved by the natural acids present in the apples, lemons and limes.

49. Gum Problems:
Coconut oil, aloe Vera
Coconut oil can be an effective gum healer and cleanser. (It's also a lot less painful than going to the

dentist.) Using aloe Vera as mouthwash can greatly improve a multitude of gum issues.

50. Hay Fever:
Nettle tea, grapes, Echinacea, honey
Nettle tea, grapes, and Echinacea have incredible anti-histamine properties so they should ease the symptoms of hay fever (runny or blocked nose, streaming eyes, sneezing etc.)

After you finish drinking the tea, you can use the teabags to calm eye irritation.

Local honey is a perfect remedy for hay fever, as it builds up the body's natural tolerance to the locally occurring flora and fauna.

51. Headache:
Chamomile tea, garlic, water
More often than not, the cause of a headache is dehydration, stress or muscle tension. If you are suffering from a headache, always insure you are drinking as much water as possible.

Raw garlic and chamomile tea can relax stressed minds and muscles. For me, the garlic removes the headache quicker than the chamomile.

52. Heartburn:
Ginger, probiotic yoghurt
My brother used to suffer terribly from heartburn. He experienced minimal to no relief from over-the-

counter heartburn medicines. While I was pregnant, all the midwives suggested ginger nut biscuits to alleviate morning sickness and heartburn.

My brother tried this and found it helped but he had to eat ginger biscuits all evening to keep it at bay. That is a lot of sugar! One day, he succumbed to a bout of heartburn. Since we had no biscuits handy, we went into a veggie shop and bought a piece of ginger root. He broke off a thumb-sized piece of ginger, crushed it with his fingers and swallowed it down with water. Within two minutes, he started professing that the pain was easing. Within five minutes, he felt fine. On top of that, probiotic yoghurts promote healthy stomach and gut functions, and prove to be a great way to prevent heartburn.

53. Hemorrhoids:
Leafy greens, oats, water
(See: Piles)

54. Hives:
Nettle tea, chamomile tea, oats, coconut oil
Hives are usually related to heat or histamine. Nettle tea and chamomile tea are the perfect antihistamine drinks to partake in when you have hives.

You can also make coconut oil and oat salve to cool the itch.

Do not use pure aloe Vera on the hives as this can spread the rash.

55. Hyperactivity:

Chamomile tea, warm milk and honey

If your child is hyperactive at night or if your own mind is overactive, try chamomile tea. It is a natural de-stresser.

Warm milk and honey works wonders at relaxing an over-active mind (especially in children.) Not only does it help you sleep but you should arise energized and refreshed.

56. Indigestion:

Probiotic yoghurt

Probiotic yoghurt encourages digestive functions, making indigestion less likely to occur.

57. Infections (Chest, Throat, Sinus):

Garlic, honey, lemon

Garlic and honey are the two most renowned natural antibiotic and anti-viral foods there are. If they are accompanied with or mixed with lemon water, they can boost the immune system and are great at countering chest, throat and sinus infections.

58. Inflammation:

Turmeric tea

Turmeric has active anti-inflammatory properties. Whether you have menstrual bloating or swollen arthritic joints, turmeric can noticeably bring down the inflammation.

59. Insomnia:
Chamomile tea, milk and honey
(See: Hyperactivity)

60. Itching:
Nettle tea, chamomile tea
Itching can be histamine-based, so these teas can quell the problem.

61. Intestinal Health:
Beans, leafy greens, oats, sweet potato, probiotic yoghurt
(See: Digestive health)
High fiber foods promote and support intestinal health.

62. Jaundice (In Babies):
Breast Milk
Mild jaundice in newborns is quite common. The absolute best thing for infant jaundice is breastfeeding. Breastfeeding provides all of the enzymes necessary to aid your baby's liver functions. If you think your baby has jaundice, always check with a doctor to assess the severity.

63. Kidney Infection:
Cranberries, water
Many people have been told to drink cranberry juice for kidney infections. While cranberries are effective,

the problem is the amount of sugar or sugar substitutes (depending on the particular brand.) It serves you better to make a cranberry smoothie.

Extra water will also help flush your kidneys out.

64. Kidney Stones:
Apples, lemon and limes
Like gallstones, several apples a day accompanied by lemon and lime water will help the body dissolve the stones.

65. Lung Infection:
Garlic, sage, water
Garlic's antibiotic qualities will help the immune system fight off infection, while breathing in sage water steam can open and cleanse the bronchioles.

66. Mastitis: (Breast inflammation)
Cabbage Leaves
When I had mastitis, the midwives suggested chilling cabbage leaves in the freezer and placing them inside the bra a couple of times a day for half an hour. This should quickly decrease the inflammation.

Be careful not to wear the leaves all day as it might diminish your milk levels.

67. Menopause:
(See: Perimenopause)

68. Menstrual Cramps:

Raspberry leaf tea, chamomile tea

Raspberry leaf tea and chamomile tea provide me almost instantaneous relief from menstrual cramps.

69. Miscarriage (After):

Raspberry Leaf tea

Since a miscarriage is still a labor, the uterus needs to recover. Just like after childbirth, raspberry leaf tea can heal the post-miscarriage uterus.

70. Mucus:

Raspberries, sage, water

Raspberries are known to expel mucus. You can take the sage steam option to soften and clear the mucus.

Drinking plenty of water will also help with clearing mucus.

71. Nausea:

Ginger, Probiotic yoghurt

Ginger is an excellent cure for nausea. Probiotic yoghurt is a milder option. It's effective because it adds good bacteria to the stomach.

72. Neuralgia:

Turmeric, garlic

Because of their anti-inflammatory properties, garlic and turmeric can reduce nerve pain.

73. Pain:
(See: Aches and Cramps)

74. Perimenopause:
Raspberry leaf tea, raspberries, pomegranate, chamomile tea, lavender tea, turmeric
Perimenopause is what most people refer to as "The Change", the time before menopause (menopause is when you haven't had a menstrual bleed for a year). At this time, your Follicle Stimulating Hormone (FSH) will raise and estrogen will decrease, both can fluctuate. These hormonal changes take place as your ovaries begin to decline in functionality. This phase can last two to ten years, (or less in the case of hysterectomy or early onset menopause.) These changes bring many symptoms. Chamomile and lavender are effective at countering anxiety or depression. Raspberries and pomegranate work for uterine health and support. Turmeric should be used for aches, cramps, headaches, etc.

75. Perspiration.
Baking soda, coconut oil, water.
Substituting coconut oil for deodorant can help with perspiration, as it is antifungal and antibacterial. Because it has less chemical density than regular deodorants, it doesn't clog the pores and sweat glands which will help to eliminate bad odors. Baking soda

absorbs moisture and neutralizes odors, making it an ideal deodorant.

Proper hydration will prevent overheating, which will lessen your body's "cool down" response.

76. Piles:
Leafy greens, oats, water
Piles are generally caused from having to bare down too hard during bowel movements. Having a high fiber, well-hydrated diet will prevent and alleviate this problem.

77. Pneumonia:
Garlic, lemon water, sage
If you are at home while suffering with pneumonia, you can add garlic, lemon water and sage steam to your regime to speed up the recovery.

78. Psoriasis:
Coconut oil
Although diet can aggravate or cause psoriasis, not every patient has the same trigger foods. Coconut oil can be used as a moisturizer when psoriasis flares up, which helps to prevent sore cracks in the affected skin. A close relative of mine suffered from psoriasis and found great relief from this oil. However, the problem continued until she got acupuncture treatment. The psoriasis has not flared up since.

79. Rash.

Coconut oil, basil oil.

When dealing with a lacey rash, (like you would get from a mild penicillin allergic reaction or measles,) mixing a couple of drops of pure basil essential oil with coconut oil will create a mild, non-irritating salve for the rash.

80. Rheumatism/Rheumatoid Arthritis;

Cayenne pepper, garlic, turmeric tea
(See: Aches)

81. Scalds:

Aloe Vera, water
(See: Burns)

Scalds are caused by boiling water or steam. This type of burn can penetrate the skin without breaking it. If you have been scalded in the hand, foot, face, or on any joints, it is best to visit a doctor to insure the injury hasn't damaged deeper than you think.

82. Sciatica:

Chamomile tea, turmeric tea

Accompany these teas with some simple back, hip and leg stretches will help work the nerve out from where it is trapped. The results can be immediate but it shouldn't take longer than a few days.

83. Shingles:

Coconut oil, oats, water

As with chicken pox, shingles is another ailment that has to run its course. The spots are very painful and itchy. Luckily, the coconut oil/oats paste can ease the itch. Oat baths are great at bringing some relief. Drink plenty of extra water to avoid dehydration and to aid the body in flushing out the virus.

84. Sinusitis:

Garlic, sage, Echinacea

Partaking in your sage steam regime will help open and clean the airways if you suffer from sinusitis.

Adding Echinacea to your regular intake will also give your immune system an extra helping hand. Hopefully, this should make you less susceptible to bacteria that sets off your sinusitis. Garlic's strong antibiotic qualities will add extra immune system support.

85. Skin:

Coconut oil

Coconut oil is the perfect friend for any skin ailment whether it is dry, oily, sensitive or cracked. It also proves effective against acne, eczema, cuts, scrapes, psoriasis, etc.

86. Sprains:

Beans/lentils, leafy greens, arnica

Consuming these foods is vital after exercise to stop you from sustaining sprains. If you have already suffered a sprain, arnica cream can be rubbed on the joint to speed up the healing process.

87.Synovitis:

Turmeric

Synovitis is the swelling of a joint membrane. Turmeric tea or smoothies are wonderful for bringing down inflammation.

88. Stye:

Teabags, Echinacea

Styes (also known as hordeolum) are sore pimple-like lumps that appear on the eyelid. They usually occur when the immune system is run down. If you place used teabags on your eyes, it can draw the infection out of the eyelid, while bringing down the swelling.

As styes are usually a sign that the immune system is lacking, Echinacea is the perfect tea to opt for.

89. Teeth:

Coconut oil

(See: Bleeding gums)

90. Throat Infection:

Garlic, grapefruit, lemon, salt water

Since grapefruit is known for healing throat infections, you should try a freshly pressed or blended grapefruit juice/smoothie or eating fresh grapefruit slices to help your throat recover. Drinking lemon water and gargling salt water provides cleansing for your throat. It also helps to get rid of viruses and bacteria. Garlic has natural antibiotic and anti-viral qualities, which is essential for throat infections.

91. Thrush:

Coconut oil, probiotic yoghurt

Whether you have oral thrush, vaginal thrush, or thrush on your nipples, coconut oil and probiotic are safe and effective. After giving birth, I had vaginal thrush numerous times. Prescribed pessaries cleared the thrush but it kept returning.

When I changed to coconut oil it cleared the thrush and it has never returned.

92. Tongue Boils:

Rock/sea salt, water

Nothing works better for a pimple or boil on the tongue than salt water. What you need to do is mix pure rock salt or sea salt with half a cup of boiling water. Allow it to cool until it is palatable and then swirl it around your mouth. Spit out and repeat until the cup is empty. This will bring immediate relief. If you act early enough, it will resolve the issue overnight.

93. Tonsillitis:
Garlic, grapefruit, lemon, salt water
(See: Throat Infection)

94. Urinary Tract Infection:
Cranberry juice, coconut oil, garlic, water
Freshly squeezed cranberry juice/smoothies will help flush your urinary tract infection.

Using coconut oil keeps redness and irritation at bay during a Urinary Tract Infection (UTI.) As with all infections, garlic is a must-have.

95. Urticaria
Nettle tea, chamomile tea, oat bath
An urticarial rash is an extreme version of hives. An urticarial rash flares up either in large patches, all over, or starting from the head and gradually working its way down the body. It is usually heat or histamine-related, so nettle tea and chamomile tea is a lifesaver.

When my son had a head-to-toe rash, the nettle tea calmed the redness and itch, and the chamomile helped him drift off to sleep.

As with any itch, your oat bath or paste will hopefully give some relief.

96. Viral Infections:

Blueberries, garlic, Echinacea

These three immune boosters are my top recommendations for any kind of ailment. You can mix all three into a smoothie and add some pressed orange juice to kick your immune system into gear.

97. Warts:

Clove oil

If you have a wart, pour or dab it with pure clove essential oil two or three times a day. When I tried this the first few times, I felt no difference so I stopped. Two or three weeks later, I noticed the wart had disappeared. Clove oil killed it from the root and the skin just repaired itself.

98. Water retention.

Water

This one sounds like an oxymoron but upping your water intake can help reduce water retention. Your body has a habit of retaining what it is not getting enough in the same way your body ends up storing bad fats when it doesn't get enough good fats. The body will retain water if it feels it's lacking.

99. Wounds:

Aloe Vera

Aloe Vera provides excellent healing properties and can be used for most external wounds.

100. Yeast Infections:
Coconut oil, probiotic yoghurt
(See: Thrush)

SECTION 3
SIMPLE RECIPES

1.Hummus

1½ cup chickpeas
¼ cup tahini
1 lemon
1 tbsp. cumin powder
1 tbsp. rock/sea salt
½ tbsp. ground mixed pepper

Put your ingredients in a blender and turn it on.
If the hummus is too thick, add a tablespoon of water and blend again.
Repeat until desired texture is reached.

2. Mint Dip

This is the easiest dip to prepare.

Mint leaves
Probiotic natural yoghurt.

Mix the two together, et voila!!
Mint dip is perfect for zucchini fritters, chips, sweet
potato fries or veg sticks.

3. Beetroot Hummus

Remove the outer layer of the beetroot and place it in aluminum foil with a drizzle of melted coconut oil.
Roast for one hour at 200°c.
Remove from oven when a knife slides into the beet easily.
Allow to cool.
While cooling, repeat the steps from your hummus recipe. **(See: Hummus)**
Now blend your roast beetroot.
Combine this with the chickpea mix and you should have delicious, vibrant, pink hummus.
Serve with coriander leaves and feta cheese crumbs, with a side of carrot/celery/bread sticks/crackers to dip.

4. Guacamole

1 avocado
½ cup spinach leaves
Juice of 1 lemon
1 tbsp. paprika
¼ tbsp. salt
¼ tbsp. pepper

Mix all ingredients, blend and serve.

5. Powerful Pesto

¼ cup of pine nuts
1 cup of basil leaves
¼ cup spinach leaves
1 tbsp. hemp seeds
1 tbsp. linseed/flaxseed
1 clove garlic
¼ tbsp. rock/sea salt
½ cup chamomile/olive oil

Blend all ingredients together, adding more oil if necessary.
Add to freshly cooked pastas, salads, on pizza etc.

6. Courgette Fritters

1 courgette/zucchini
1 large carrot
1 large potato

Grate all of your ingredients into a bowl.
Season the ingredients with salt and pepper.
Scoop them out and mold them into flat patties.
Fry them until they are browned on either side.
Serve with mint dip.

7. Crackers

2 tbsp. chia seeds
2 tbsp. linseed/flaxseed
½ cup crushed cashew nuts
½ cup pumpkin seeds
¼ cup sunflower seeds
¼ cup hemp seeds
½ tbsp. dry rosemary
½ tbsp. dry oregano
1 cup coconut flour
½ tbsp. rock/sea salt
¼ tbsp. ground pepper
1 cup of milk

Mix dry ingredients in a mixing bowl, then add milk and mix well.
Line a baking tray with greaseproof paper, and spread your mixture evenly and thinly (but not too thin. About 1cm.)
Bake at 200°c for 15-20 mins.
Remove from oven, flip cracker and cut into as many smaller crackers as you like. Return to oven and bake for a further 15-20 mins.
When the crackers begin to curl at the edges slightly, they are done.
Cool on a wire rack and then store in an airtight container.

8. Vegetable Soup

2 tbsp. coconut oil
1 large onion
2 cloves of garlic
1 thumb-sized piece of ginger
2 stalks of celery
Pinch of salt and pepper
500mls water
Potatoes, carrots, sweet potato, broccoli, cauliflower
or whatever veg you have in the fridge that will fill ¾
a medium (2l) saucepan when chopped

Wash, peel and chop all of your vegetables.
Melt the coconut oil in your saucepan on a medium
heat.
Add the onion, garlic, ginger, and celery.
Allow it to fry for 3 mins.
Add your chopped veg, blanching them (Frying) in
the coconut oil mix, locking in all the flavor.
Finally, add the water, salt and pepper, put a lid on
and allow to simmer away for 20 mins.
Now you're ready to blend and serve.

9. Carrot and Coriander Soup

1 tbsp. of coconut oil
1 large onion
2 cloves garlic
Thumb-sized piece of ginger
1 tbsp. cumin powder
1 tbsp. coriander powder
Pinch of salt and pepper
500mls water
8-10 med-large carrots

Firstly, melt the coconut oil in a saucepan over a medium heat.
Add the cumin, coriander powders, garlic, ginger and onion.
Fry for 3 mins.
Next, add your carrots, blanching them in the coconut oil mix.
Finally, add salt, pepper and water, cover with a lid and allow to simmer for 20 minutes.
Blend and serve.

10. Super Salad

Spinach leaves
Rocket leaves
Red lettuce leaves
Coriander/cilantro leaves
Parsley leaves
Basil leaves
1 red pepper
1 yellow pepper
Black and green olives
Spring onions
Chives (including purple flower head)
Tomatoes
Olive oil
1 med carrot
½ cucumber
Honey
Mozzarella

Wash and prepare ingredients. (I like to chop all my ingredients into long but thin strips. The only exceptions are the carrots and cucumber. I prefer to have them grated over all of my leaves.)
Insert all of the leaves in a large salad bowl.
Next, add your tomatoes, peppers, chives and onions, topping it with grated carrot and cucumber.
Now, drizzle the olive oil and honey over the top.
Add the mozzarella to finish.

11. Pilau Rice

4 crushed cardamom pods
5 bay leaves
4 cloves
½ tbsp. turmeric
1/3 tsp fennel seeds
1 cup basmati rice

Melt coconut oil in a saucepan over a medium heat.
Lightly fry spices and seeds.
Add cup of rice, fry for 2 mins.
Pour in two cups of water.
Boil the water and then turn the heat down low and
cover pot with lid, leaving a slight opening to allow
steam to leave the pot.
Do not stir, allow water to evaporate, remove bay
leaves and then it is ready to serve.

12. Porridge Bread

1 500ml tub of probiotic yoghurt
2 x 500ml tub full of porridge oats
2 pinches of salt
1 tbsp. baking powder

In a large mixing bowl, mix your dry ingredients.
Then add your yoghurt.
Mix thoroughly.
Pour mixture into a loaf tin.
Bake at 200°c for 30 mins approx.
Allow it to cool in tin.
Remove when tin is cool to touch.
Place bread on wire rack and cover with a tea towel as it finishes cooling.

13. Sweet Potato Fries

1 med sweet potato per person

Peel and chip sweet potato
Place on non-stick baking tray.
Drizzle oil (or melted butter if you're feeling naughty.)
Season with salt and pepper.
Bake for 25 mins at 200°c.

14. Kulcha Bread

3 cups (400g) flour
1/3 tbsp. baking soda
½ tbsp. baking powder
1 pinch sugar
1 tbsp. salt
Pinch of black pepper
1 tbsp. oil (olive/chamomile/rapeseed oil)
2 tbsp. probiotic natural yoghurt

Pour dry mix in a bowl.
In a separate bowl, mix yoghurt and oil.
Add wet mix to dry mix, mixing together until it
becomes doughy.
Knead for 5 mins, cover bowl and leave. (You can use
the dough after half an hour, but 1-2 hours is best; 1
hour in a hot kitchen, 2 in a cool kitchen.)
Break into balls, flatten, fry in a non-stick pan until
raised slightly and browned, or alternatively bake in
oven.
Put on greaseproof paper on a baking tray until raised
slightly and browned.

15. Simple Indian Style Dinner

1 can chickpeas/500g soaked chickpeas
1 med sweet potato
1 can aduki/kidney beans
1 handful of spinach
1 large onion
2 cloves of garlic
1 inch of ginger
½ tsp coriander/cilantro powder
½ tbsp. cumin powder
½ tbsp. turmeric powder
½ tbsp. garam masala powder
pinch of salt and pepper
1 ½ tbsp. Coconut oil

Start by peeling and chopping all of your fresh
ingredients to your preferred size.
Heat the coconut oil in a shallow frying pan on a
medium heat.
Add the spices first, frying them until they become
paste-like.
Add your onions, garlic and ginger.
Let them fry for 1 min.
Add the rest of the ingredients.
Stir them and make sure everything is coated with the
spicy oil.
Place a lid on top, and allow it to fry for 10-15 mins
on medium heat, stirring occasionally.

Add the spinach for the last 3 mins.
You can serve this alone or with a portion of brown rice or pilau rice.

16. Vegetable Korma

100g quinoa
1 can chickpeas
2 medium potatoes
2 large carrots
½ aubergine (zucchini)
½ courgette (eggplant)
Garlic
½ onion
1 thumb of ginger
Peppers
Coconut oil

Peel and chop everything finely.
Heat oil in a pan, first frying garlic, onions, ginger, and peppers.
Next add veg and fry until softened and browned slightly.

For the sauce;
½ onion
Clove of garlic
Thumb of ginger
1tbsp. turmeric
1tbsp. garam masala
½ tbsp. mild chili powder
½ tbsp. cumin powder
6 tbsp. natural probiotic yoghurt

In a saucepan on a medium heat, melt the
coconut oil.
Fry garlic and ginger.
Next add spices, fry for 2 mins.
Add yoghurt and mix.
If it doesn't look enough for the veg, just add a
couple more scoops of yoghurt.

Mix sauce into veg and cook for a further 15-20 mins.
Serve with rice or kulcha bread.

17. Fake-Away Pizza

For the Base:
1 1/3 cup of flour (any flour of your choosing;
coconut, whole meal, even organic white flour will be
better than anything from the take away or
supermarket freezer.)
¼ tbsp. of sea salt/pink Himalayan rock salt
1 pinch mixed ground pepper
½ tbsp. gluten free baking powder (I have forgotten
the baking powder on a few occasions and it has
made no difference to the final outcome so if you
have none, go for it.)
1/3 cup milk
1 ½ tbsp. of chamomile/olive/ground nut
oil/Sunflower/chamomile/olive oil

Mix all your dry ingredients in a mixing bowl.
Then pour the milk over.
Add the oil.
Mix and knead until you get a smooth, doughy
consistency.
You may need a tiny splash of milk if it's too floury,
or an extra pinch or two of flour if its sticky.
Place bowl over the dough for 10 mins.
While the dough sits, you can make your sauce.

For the Sauce:

This makes enough for two pizzas. It can be kept in the fridge for three or four days in an airtight tub, and can be used for pastas also.

1 tin chopped tomatoes
1 pinch fresh chopped basil leaves
1 pinch fresh chopped coriander/cilantro leaves
1 pinch fresh chopped parsley leaves
¼ tbsp. sea salt/pink Himalayan rock salt
1 tbsp. chamomile/olive/ground nut oil
2 med cloves garlic

Dried herb leaves will do if you don't have fresh herbs. However, fresh herbs will give you a richer flavor.

Pop all in a blender, blend until smooth, a voila! Pizza sauce.

Next, roll your dough to your chosen shape and size. The bigger you go, the thinner the base will be, so I roll it out big.

Place atop grease paper on a baking tray.

Bake the base at 200°c for 6 mins.

Take it out and then add your sauce and toppings of your choice.

Return to oven for 15-20 mins.

18. Dahl

200g red split lentils
½ tbsp. mustard seeds
Thumb of ginger
1 tbsp. hing/asafoetida
1 tbsp. garam masala
1 tbsp. turmeric
1 tbsp. cumin seeds

Boil water and then add lentils.
Keep the lentils in the water for about 15 mins until they are swollen and soft. Periodically, remove the scum that comes to the top.
Once cooked, strain out the water.

In a frying pan/skillet, dry fry your cumin seeds, crush and put aside.
Melt your oil and fry your spices and seeds.
Add your lentils, fry for a further 5 mins and serve with rice.

19. Stir Fry

Noodles (any kind)
1 tbsp. coconut oil
1 clove of garlic
1 med onion
¼ red pepper
1 small sweet potato
1 large carrot
½ aubergine (eggplant)
1 medium courgette (zucchini)
1 handful of spinach
1 handful of kale
1 can of chickpeas or kidney beans (or both)
Soy sauce
Balsamic vinegar

Boil your noodles.
Steam your kale and spinach for 10 mins or until it has softened.
Fry garlic, ginger, onion, and peppers in the pan.
Add in veg.
Fry until softened.
Next add the noodles, kale and spinach.
Pour soy sauce and balsamic vinegar over it all and mix together, frying for a further 2 mins.

20. Frittata

3 eggs
1 med courgette/zucchini
1 large potato
1 large carrot
Mint leaves

Boil or steam the potatoes and carrots for 10 mins.
Mix eggs, a splash of milk, a pinch of salt and pepper in a bowl.
Finely chop the courgette.
Place all the veg and mint leaves in a small casserole dish.
Pour in the egg mix and bake for 35 mins at 200°c.

21. Chickpea Cookies

1 can chickpeas (15oz)
½ cup Natural Peanut butter
1/3 cup maple syrup
1 Vanilla pod (or 1 tbsp. extract)
¼ tbsp. rock/sea salt
½ cup choc chips

Blend or mash the chickpeas.
Pour the chickpeas into a large mixing bowl, adding all the other ingredients, keeping a ¼ cup of chocolate chips.
Line a baking tray with greaseproof paper.
Place the mix on the baking tray in cookie sized blobs (about 1 tbsp.), leaving about an inch between each blob.
Add the last of the choc chip to the top of each blob.
Bake at 180°c for 40 mins or until the cookies are golden brown and crispy at the edges.
Allow to cool on the tray for 10 mins.
Then move to a wire rack for added crunchiness.
Store in an airtight container for three or four days.

SMOOTHIES

Smoothies are a wonderful source of easily digestible nutrients, but often we just don't know what combinations will taste nice. It is important to note that smoothies should be consumed within 15 mins because oxygen removes the nutrients after 15 mins. To give you a kick start, here's my 10 favorite smoothies. With each smoothie, insert approximately a handful of each ingredient (unless specified otherwise) and a tablespoon measurement for seeds. Each recipe makes enough for a family of four.

1. Pale Yellow

Kale
Walnuts
1 orange
1 banana
1 apple
2 tbsp. turmeric powder
1tbsp. honey
Sunflower seeds
Orange juice to blend

2. Pastel Green

Kale
Spinach
Raspberries
A pear
A banana
Water to blend

3. Cream

Spinach
1 bananas
1 med carrot
Strawberries
Raspberries
Brazil nuts
Hemp seeds
Water to blend

4. Lilac

Raspberries
Blueberries
Strawberries
1 banana
Almond nuts
Sunflower seeds
Water to blend

5. Red

1 small beetroot
1 banana
Black grapes
Green grapes
Strawberries
Goji berries
Cranberry juice to blend

6. Purple

1 banana
1 small avocado
Blueberries
1 tbsp. probiotic yoghurt
Hemp seeds
Chia seeds
Cashew nuts
Water to blend

7. Orange

2 med carrots
1 orange
½ cucumber
1 peach
Strawberries
Orange juice to blend

8. Fuchsia

1 small beetroot
2 bananas
Aloe Vera (gel straight from the plant)
Water to blend
Orange juice to blend

9. Dark Green

Spinach
Kale
1 banana
1 tbsp. probiotic yoghurt
1 tbsp. spirulina powder
Cranberry juice to blend

10. Pastel Pink

1 apple
1 orange
Strawberries
Blueberries
A thumb of ginger
1 tbsp. probiotic yoghurt
Water to blend